Coffee Break in a 12-Hour Shift

2-Minute Devotional Thoughts for Healthcare Professionals on the Go

31 Days at His Feet

By

Gladys Jusino

Table of Contents

Introduction 5

Day 1 – The Gift of Compassion 8

Day 2 – The Power of Listening 10

Day 3 – Gratitude in Everyday Life 12

Day 4 – Fortress Amid Chaos 14

Day 5 – Nurturing Our Purpose 16

Day 6 – The Importance of Community 18

Day 7 – Renewed Hope 20

Day 8 – Strength in Weakness 22

Day 9 – Wisdom in Decision-Making 24

Day 10 – The Value of Rest 26

Day 11 – The Joy of Service 28

Day 12 – Light in Darkness 30

Day 13 – The Importance of Gratitude 32

Day 14 – Finding Purpose in Suffering 34

Day 15 – The Renewal of the Mind 36

Day 16 – Goodness of the Heart 38

Day 17 – Inner Peace 40

Day 18 – Hope in Adversity 42

Day 19 – The Joy of the Soul 44

Day 20 – Joy in Small Actions 46

Day 21 – Service: A Shared Gift 48

Day 22 – Humility in Service 50
Day 23 – The Echo of Generosity 52
Day 24 – The Art of Being Present 54
Day 25 – Pause as a Sacred Act 56
Day 26 – Rest amid Service 58
Day 27 – Leaving Burdens in God's Hands 60
Day 28 – Renewing the Vocation from Stillness 62
Day 29 – Ever-Present Faithfulness 64
Day 30 – His Presence in Every Breath 66
Day 31 – Grace for Every Step 68

Introduction

The Journey of Healthcare Professionals: Finding Balance

Healthcare professionals face the ongoing challenge of balancing the care they provide for others with their well-being. Years ago, a friend would call me in the middle of a 12-hour shift every time she felt anxiety sneaking in. We would go to the locker room, hold hands, and do breathing exercises. That would calm her down, and she would be able to complete the rest of the shift. As a Christian, I should have prayed with her to help her understand that "anxiety develops when we try to do things by ourselves, instead of letting God take care of things." In those days, I couldn't understand why she got so anxious.

Today, I understand completely why. I attended church daily during my upbringing. Yes. As a family, we were involved in everything. Life was good and quiet, and that was the norm. Recently, I have been hearing the Word as if it is the very first time, and my life has changed. Scriptural passages I have read many times are now clarifying God's purpose for humanity. It is now that my life has turned from good and quiet to a constant turmoil. In recent days, I leave my house in spiritual content and peace only to face a challenging atmosphere at work. *"For our struggle is not against flesh and blood, but against the rulers, against the authorities, against the powers of this dark world and against the spiritual forces of evil in the heavenly realms." Ephesians 6:12* I had to understand that it is not people who create the turmoil; it is the devil using people to interrupt our peace and connection with God.

I never needed to step out of the area to reconnect with God. Now, at the end of my professional career, this is a constant need; however, it is a luxury I cannot enjoy. Then, I was reminded: *"Be still and know that I am God." Psalm 46:10*

Amid the constant movement and demands of caring for others, true peace can be found in brief pauses where we deliberately seek God's presence. When we quiet our minds, even for a moment, we create space for the Spirit to renew our strength. These moments, whether a silent breath, a glance at the sky, or a whispered prayer, remind us that God dwells with us in every corner of our day, offering repose, hope, and sustaining grace. Let each moment of stillness be an invitation to trust, rest, and remember that we are never alone.

This devotional book is designed to offer a brief, 2-minute pause each day—a chance for reflection. This book aims to help healthcare professionals renew their spirit and reconnect with God. A 2-minute break allows you to reset your mind and be in tune with God's Spirit, able to carry on. I hope the words shared in this book foster balance and inner peace in your life as you continue to labor in this world until Jesus' return.

How to Use this Book

Face it. You need to step outside of the chaos and reconnect with God. That is the only way to create balance within your soul. Any workplace offers its employees a 15-minute break. Take it and be intentional about using it to break away from the negativity, chaos, and dysfunction that can occasionally be found in the workplace. Sit in a quiet place. Upon opening this book, readers will find guidance for their professional purpose and the intended role within healthcare as informed by Christian principles. Each day features a Bible verse, accompanied by a concise reflection and prayer. The intention is for those words to become a balm to your soul and a guide to face daily challenges with serenity and hope. There are project and practice ideas connected to some of the devotionals. Use those ideas to foster qualities and practices presented in the devotionals, as needed. Keep a journal to write any insights God places in your heart as you sit still and quiet and let Him share His heart with you. May you find spiritual comfort and peace throughout these 31 days at His feet.

Day 1 – The Gift of Compassion

"Blessed are the merciful, for they will receive mercy." – Matthew 5:7

Compassion is at the heart of our profession. Think of moments when someone showed compassion towards you. How was it demonstrated, and how did it feel? Now, think of ways in which you can show compassion not only to your patients but also to yourself. Practicing self-compassion is essential for maintaining resilience and preventing burnout, which enables us to support those who rely on us. Taking time to be gentle with yourself is not a luxury, but a necessity. Allow yourself to receive the same kindness you extend to others. Recognize your own needs and nurture them with patience and understanding. Self-compassion fortifies your spirit. It enables you to serve with renewed energy and a full heart. Remember, you cannot pour from an empty cup. Embrace moments of rest, reflection, and gratitude as gifts to yourself, and let your soul be replenished by the grace and love that you so generously give to others.

Lord, help me to be compassionate to others and myself. Fill my heart with your love and allow that love to be reflected throughout this day in my actions, words, and thoughts.

PROJECT IDEA

Volunteer for Disaster Relief Assistance

When disaster hits, it takes a lot to help rebuild a community. In partnership with an emergency relief organization, raise money, volunteer your time to conduct health assessments for those affected, or organize supply drives to help those affected by natural disasters. (Boterra.com)

Day 2 – The Power of Listening

"Everyone who is wise in heart accepts the commandments, but the fool in his lips will be punished." – Proverbs 10:8

True listening is an act of humility. When we pay attention to what others are saying, without judgment, we allow the other person to feel seen and valued. Listening with intention cultivates an atmosphere of trust and compassion. Listening with intention brings healing not only physically but also emotionally and spiritually. As healthcare professionals, our ability to listen to others can transform patient care, creating a space where individuals feel understood and supported. Before each interaction, remind yourself of the gift of presence you are about to offer, and notice how this simple act of listening can bring peace and understanding to your interactions. Listening will enrich life and the lives of those you serve.

God, give me an attentive heart and ears willing to listen. Father, show me the reason why I have been chosen to hear what others have to say. May I be an instrument of your peace by welcoming those around me with understanding and empathy.

PROJECT IDEA

Donate Your Time at a Soup Kitchen

If you're known for your talents in the kitchen, share your favorite meals with those who need them most in your local soup kitchen. Not the handiest with the stove? Feel free to drop by and lend a hand, serving warm meals to your low-income and homeless neighbors. Take the time to communicate with the participants and **hear** their stories.

Day 3 – Gratitude in Everyday Life

"Give thanks in everything, for this is the will of God for you in Christ Jesus."
– Thessalonians 5:18

Gratitude transforms the way we experience life. It is not easy to see the good when you are surrounded by darkness. Today, look for reasons, even small ones, to be thankful: a smile, a kind word, the opportunity to serve. Gratitude opens the door to genuine joy and contentment. Please take a moment to acknowledge your environment and the positive aspects present in your current situation. When you cultivate gratitude in your heart, even the most challenging days can be transformed into opportunities for growth and peace. Share gratitude with others to help build a kinder world.

Lord, help me to recognize your blessings in everyday life. May my heart remain grateful in difficult times. God, open my eyes to see what you want me to see.

PRACTICE IDEA

Count Your Daily Blessings

Before bed or when you wake up, take a few minutes to name three things you are grateful for within yourself, and then three things that are more external, either big or small. As you pause to acknowledge these aspects, you may find a renewed sense of peace and contentment, setting a positive tone for the day or aiding in a restful night's sleep. Reflecting on internal attributes, such as your resilience, creativity, or kindness, helps build self-compassion. Recognizing external blessings, like the beauty of nature, the support of loved ones, or a comforting cup of tea, cultivates a broader sense of gratitude. Over time, this habit can enhance your overall well-being, encouraging you to notice and cherish the abundance in your life.

Day 4 – Fortress Amid Chaos

"The Lord gives strength to his people; the Lord blesses his people with peace."
– Psalm 29:11

At times, life and the healthcare environment can feel overwhelming. True strength comes not just from our efforts but from trusting God's control. Relying solely on others can lead to deception. Take a moment to pause and embrace peace that surpasses understanding. In the quietness of that moment, allow yourself to feel the gentle reassurance that comes from trusting the One who is greater than yourself. Remember that it is not the circumstances around you that define your peace, but the steadfast presence of God within you. True peace is not the absence of challenges, but the presence of divine assurance amid them. May this peace anchor you, bringing calm and wisdom to every decision you face.

Father, in chaos and haste, grant me serenity. Allow me to see you at work in the background, as I continue to do what I must do. May I find in you the refuge and calm to continue serving with dedication and hope, regardless of what happens around me.

PRACTICE IDEA

Read a Book

Some books can help you transform your life, strengthening your faith. Some ideas are: *Speak Out God's Promises Over Your Life*, by Joseph Prince; *Help is Here: Finding Fresh Strength and Purpose in the Power of the Holy Spirit*, by Max Lucado; *Strength in the Struggle: A Bible Study Workbook for Women on Letting Go of Fear and Anxiety*, by Lauren Ibach.

Day 5 – Nurturing Our Purpose

"For I know the plans that I have for you, says the Lord, plans of prosperity and not of calamity, to give you a future and a hope." – Jeremiah 29:11

Keeping the passion and a sense of purpose alive strengthens our spirit. Today, reflect on what led you to dedicate yourself to caring for others. Let that purpose be revitalized within you and propel you onward. Remember the moments when you first felt called to serve, the experiences that ignited your passion, and motivated you to make a difference in the lives of others. These memories are not just remnants of the past; they are sparks that can reignite your dedication and remind you of the profound impact you have on those around you. Embracing the joy and fulfillment that comes from knowing your work is not just a job, but a mission filled with meaning and compassion.

God, renew in me the desire to serve and the clarity of my purpose, and reveal your plan for me in this position I am in. May every day be an opportunity to honor your calling on my life.

PROJECT IDEA

Host Workshops for Students and Other Healthcare Professionals

Workshops serve as an essential resource, aiding healthcare professionals and students in enhancing their knowledge and skills while also pinpointing areas for improvement. Organize a workshop or host one yourself to help healthcare professionals develop their skills and foster better patient care.

Day 6 – The Importance of Community

"Two are better than one, because they are better paid for their work."
– Ecclesiastes 4:9

We are not meant to walk alone. We find support, encouragement, and comfort in the company of others. Building connections and working together can help make daily responsibilities more manageable. In the journey of life, community becomes a sanctuary where we gather strength and solace. It is within this fellowship that we discover the power of unity, where joys are multiplied and sorrows are divided. Each interaction offers an opportunity to uplift and be uplifted, to listen and be heard. Think of those who have supported you and thank them for the value they bring to your life. Allow your interactions to reflect warmth and sincerity, whether through kindness or shared silence.

Lord, thank you for the people you put in my path. May I offer support to those around me and accept assistance when needed with humility.

PROJECT IDEA

Mentor Young Professionals

Mentorship programs offer significant benefits for older teens and young adults, providing them with practical experience, personalized guidance, and the opportunity to forge relationships that will pave the way for their career success. (Boterratech.com) Through mentorship, young individuals can develop essential skills such as critical thinking, communication, and problem-solving, which are crucial in today's dynamic work environment. The bonds formed in these programs often lead to long-lasting professional networks that continue to support both mentors and mentees throughout their careers. Ultimately, mentorship serves as a bridge connecting academic learning with real-world applications, enriching the personal and professional lives of everyone involved.

Day 7 – Renewed Hope

"Those who place their hope in the Lord will find their strength renewed; they will soar on wings like eagles, they will run without becoming weary, and they will walk without tiring." – Isaiah 40:31

Hope is the engine that drives us to keep going even on difficult days. Allow yourself today to renew your hopes and trust that every day is a new opportunity to grow and serve with love. Ask God to reveal what He wants you to focus on in your day and find renewed hope in chaos. Every day brings the promise of a fresh start, filled with endless possibilities. During those moments of quiet reflection, let your heart be open to the whispers of God's word. Let God guide you, showing you the path forward. As you face daily challenges, remember that hope is a constant anchor for your soul. Find strength in the knowledge that each step you take is guided by God's loving hand. May your renewed hope inspire others around you to seek the light of God in their journeys.

Father, renew my hope. May I never lack confidence in your promises and the desire to continue growing under your guidance.

PRACTICE IDEA

Steps to Renew Hope

Acknowledge that you have lost hope or that hope is slipping away. Rest. Jesus pulled away from the crowds and demands of life. Read the Bible. A chapter of the Bible can give you the wisdom you need for that day, calming your spirit. Surround yourself with people who can offer words of wisdom about how faith in Christ brings goodness to your life. Claim your *Ebenezers* (1 Samuel 7:12). Find ways to mark occasions and remember the times in life that the Lord helped you.

Day 8 – Strength in Weakness

"My grace is sufficient for you, for my power is made perfect in weakness."
– 2 Corinthians 12:9

Sometimes, we feel that our strength is weakening and that we cannot move forward. It is in those moments when God's grace is most clearly manifested. Recognize your weaknesses and allow God to sustain you. Remember that everything you are and have comes from God. It is not about you, but about the One who lives in you. Acknowledge your vulnerabilities as opportunities for growth and transformation. Allow those weaknesses to deepen your reliance on God's strength. Through God's grace, you find purpose and resilience in times of weakness. Let this understanding bring peace to your heart, knowing that you are part of a greater plan, woven together by God's love and wisdom. Reflect on the ways God's presence has uplifted you in times of need, turning challenges into triumphs.

Heavenly Father, in my moments of weakness, I ask you to be my strength. Help me to remember that in You, I find everything I need to overcome any challenge. In those moments, be my high tower, my shield, and my refuge.

PRACTICE IDEA

Embracing the Journey of Growth

Identify a weakness, why you want to improve it, and your expected outcome. Set a SMART goal. Track your progress through self-assessment and peer feedback. Find models and mentors who have mastered the weakness you wish to develop. Go to them directly. Make mistakes and learn from them. Mistakes are part of the learning journey, and you can use them as opportunities for growth.

Day 9 – Wisdom in Decision-Making

"If any of you lacks wisdom, ask God for it, and he will give it to you."
– James 1:5

Every day, our decisions shape our lives and impact those around us. Relying on God's wisdom guides us to act wisely and compassionately, knowing we are not alone in our choices. Allow yourself to listen in silence to the voice of wisdom that God offers and walk with serenity before each choice. May your decisions be guided by a heart aligned with His teachings. By allowing this in your heart, a spirit of kindness and understanding will be revealed in every interaction. Each choice is an opportunity to reflect God's love and compassion in the world. Embrace each moment with gratitude. Let your actions be a testament to the divine wisdom that dwells within you and move forward with confidence and grace. Let the wisdom of God illuminate your mind, bringing clarity and peace to each step you take.

Lord, enlighten my mind and heart when I make decisions. Give me clarity to discern your will and always act with humility and generosity.

PRACTICE IDEA

Discernment Exercise

Name a complex decision you must make in your life. Commit to engage in two or three practices per week, for four weeks: Pray regularly for guidance, Journal weekly about your learning, Read the Bible, Share your decision with a small group, and have them offer their insights, Share the decision with friends and family, and have them ask you difficult questions and pray for you, Research, Meet with a trusted friend once a week to check in. (Faithlead.org)

Day 10 – The Value of Rest

"Come unto me, all ye that labor and are heavy laden, and I will give you rest." – Matthew 11:28

Rest is essential for our physical, emotional, and spiritual well-being. Although our job demands a lot from us, we must remember the importance of resting and renewing our energies. Take a moment to recharge your spirit and be in tune with God. Step back and breathe deeply. During your busy schedule, find a moment to disconnect from the demands and reconnect with the source of your strength: God's grace. Rest is not a sign of weakness, but a necessary step to maintain the vitality needed to continue serving with love and dedication. It is only when we are intentional in creating these moments with God that we will approach each new day with renewed vigor and joy. Ask God to guide you to listen to His voice in the silence and to trust in His guidance as you serve with a heart full of compassion and grace.

Lord, teach me to find the balance between work and rest. God, grant me the wisdom to know when to stop and seek refuge in your peace.

PRACTICE IDEA

Slow Down and S.T.O.P.

When you are in your head and need a moment to pause, stop thinking about whatever is in your current train of thought and redirect it healthily. Body Response: This practice physically stops the body and mind in their tracks, allowing you to regain confidence in your experience and take a refreshing breath, engaging the parasympathetic nervous system.

S: Stop what you are doing

T: Take a breath

O: Observe your surroundings

P: Peacefully proceed

Day 11 – The Joy of Service

"There is more joy in giving than in receiving." – Acts 20:35

Our work can be tiring at times, yet it offers us the chance to give and serve others. Approach each act of service with professionalism, recognizing the positive influence you have on both patients and colleagues. Each act of kindness is a gift to both the giver and the receiver. True fulfillment arises when you pour your heart out in service, knowing your small gestures can uplift and inspire others. Let every task, no matter how routine, become an opportunity to sow compassion and grace, because these moments light up the lives of those around you. In your service, discover a wellspring of happiness that flourishes not in recognition but in the quiet satisfaction of making a difference. Approach each day with a spirit of generosity, and you will find that the joy of serving never ceases to renew your soul.

God, fill my heart with joy in service. Each day presents a chance to share your love and compassion with those who need it the most. May my life reflect a life of joy, no matter the circumstances.

PROJECT IDEA

Support Prison Reentry Programs

Formerly incarcerated individuals face many challenges when reintegrating into society. By offering support through technology classes, resume workshops, or interview clothing drives, we can help these individuals start their new lives with confidence. (Boterratech.com)

Day 12 – Light in Darkness

"The Lord is my light and my salvation; whom shall I fear?" – Psalm 27:1

In times of uncertainty and darkness, remember that God is your light. Allow the clarity of His wisdom to illuminate your paths and guide you in every decision. Don't forget that you become a torch of His character wherever you might be. Be the light that guides others in purpose, direction, and clarity. Shine as a beacon of positivity when shadows gather, illuminating hope for yourself and those around you. Let your actions reflect the gentle brilliance of faith, offering warmth and comfort to hearts looking for direction. Even when the way seems uncertain, trust that your light is rooted in God's grace and can dissipate fear, revealing the path ahead. May your presence reflect God's lasting light, guiding others toward peace and assurance in every season.

Lord, be my light in the darkness. Guide my steps and help me trust your direction, even when I can't see the path clearly before me.

PROJECT IDEA

Supporting Suicide Prevention

Helping others in crisis is a noble way to contribute to your community. Volunteer to answer calls on a suicide prevention hotline to lend your ear to those in crisis and make a difference. (Boterratech.com)

Day 13 – The Importance of Gratitude

"Give thanks in all things, for this is the will of God for you in Christ Jesus."
– 1 Thessalonians 5:18

Gratitude transforms our hearts and our perspective, granting us a new direction from the situations that surround us. Ordinary moments turn into sacred gifts when our eyes are opened to the hidden blessings woven throughout each day. When we choose thankfulness, even in the middle of hardship, we invite peace and contentment to dwell within us. A grateful heart radiates warmth, uplifting not only our spirit but also those around us, inspiring hope and strength in the journey ahead. Make a list of the things you are grateful for today and allow that feeling of gratitude to fill you with peace.

God, I thank You for all the blessings You have poured into my life. Help me to maintain a grateful heart, even in the middle of difficulties.

PROJECT IDEA

Gratitude Jar

A gratitude jar serves as a powerful tool for capturing and reflecting on the positive aspects of life. Writing down things you are grateful for on small slips of paper and placing them in a jar every day will help instill a daily ritual of practicing gratitude. Engage your coworkers in this practice at your workplace. At the end of the week or month, reading through the slips of paper will help provide a reminder of the positives, fostering unity and an overall environment of gratitude in your workplace.

Day 14 – Finding Purpose in Suffering

"And we know that all things work together for good to those who love God."
– Romans 8:28

Suffering can be difficult to understand, but in every challenge, there is an opportunity to grow and find purpose. Trust that God has a plan even in the darkest of times. When trials seem overwhelming, adversity can be the soil where resilience and compassion take root. Each hardship holds the possibility to deepen your trust in God. Suffering can shape you into someone who reflects His grace more fully. When storms arise, decide to seek purpose in the process, believing that even pain can be transformed into growth and blessing. Be confident that through every hardship, God is weaving a story of redemption and hope.

Lord, help me to find purpose in suffering and to trust in your plan for my life. Strengthen my faith and allow me to see your blessings amid trials.

PRACTICE IDEA

Read a Book

The Purpose Driven Life, by Rick Warren, provides a "biblical perspective on the reason for human existence. The book asserts that your life has profound significance—God intentionally created you with a specific purpose and calling for his glory." Highlight important truths learned through the reading of this book. Create a presentation with key points that inspired you to reflect deeply on the essence of purpose and meaning. In creating the presentation, consider incorporating personal reflections and how these insights have influenced your own life journey. Using quotes from the book can also enhance the presentation's impact, offering a direct connection to the text's wisdom.

Day 15 – The Renewal of the Mind

"Do not be conformed to this world, but be transformed by the renewing of your mind." – Romans 12:2

Our mind needs to be constantly renewed to align with God's will. Take time for reflection and prayer to allow God to transform your thinking and guide you in your actions. Set aside moments each day for quiet contemplation, inviting God to shape your thoughts and renew your spirit. Through prayer and reflection, open your heart to God's guidance, allowing your mind to be refreshed and your actions to be led by grace.

Lord, renew my mind and transform my heart. Help me to think and act according to your will and to be a witness to your love in my daily work.

PRACTICE IDEA

Read an article

Move the Body, Renew the Mind: A Christian Use for Exercise, by David Mathis https://www.desiringgod.org/articles/move-the-body-renew-the-mind

Day 16 – Goodness of the Heart

"Be kind and compassionate to one another and forgiving one another."

– Ephesians 4:32

Kindness is a virtue that we must cultivate every day. When your actions reflect kindness and compassion, you will experience a transformation in your relationships and the environment. Practice forgiveness as a daily offering. Each time you choose to release resentment, you open a path for healing and unity to flourish. By letting go of past hurts, you make room for peace, understanding, and deeper relationships, allowing God's love to flow more freely through you. You will experience a clear and light environment because your heart is no longer carrying the heavy burden of past hurts. Forgiveness is not always easy, but it reflects a heart in tune with grace.

God, help me to be kind and compassionate in all my interactions. Let me reflect on your love and grace through my actions.

PROJECT IDEA

Assist A Senior Citizens Center

Building relationships across generations is important. Volunteer at a senior citizen center to get to know the older adults in your community, assist, and even make a few more friends. (Boterratech.com) Sharing stories and experiences across generations offers valuable insights and fosters a sense of community, combating loneliness for all involved. Learning about history firsthand, gaining new skills, and discovering shared interests bridge age gaps. Organizing intergenerational activities, such as art classes or gardening projects, further strengthens these bonds.

Day 17 – Inner Peace

"Peace, I leave with you; my peace I give to you; I do not give it to you as the world gives it." – John 14:27

The peace that God offers us is unlike any other. Make time to sit at the Master's feet for meditation and prayer to find that peace that surpasses all understanding and strengthens you in times of stress and anxiety. When life's winds howl and uncertainties surround you, seek refuge in the quiet assurance of God's presence. In the stillness and silent moment, let your heart be calmed and your spirit be anchored in divine peace. Invite serenity to inhabit your soul, trusting that God's gentle guidance will lead you safely through every storm and toward the tranquility that remains beyond circumstance.

Lord, give me your peace in the middle of the storms of life. Help me to trust in you and rest in your love and protection.

PRACTICE IDEA

Start a Collection

Search for Bible verses and quotes that talk about inner peace. Type them and paste them into colored index cards. In a small photo album, insert the verses. Using letter patterns, paste the word **Peace** on the album cover. Review that collection often, especially when you feel discouraged. You can include verses used in the Sunday Service that have touched on the topic of peace. This activity can be expanded by choosing other topics.

Day 18 – Hope in Adversity

"But those who wait for the Lord will have new strength; they will lift with wings like eagles." – Isaiah 40:31

Hope is the anchor of the soul. Face adversity with the assurance that God renews your strength and sustains you through every trial. When faced with uncertainty, rely on faith. Hold onto hope, trusting that the gentle hand of God will guide you through shadows and uncertainty toward new strength and courage. In times of trouble, remember that resilience flourishes in hearts anchored in God's promises. Each test is an invitation to soar above adversity, renewed and uplifted by God's steadfast faithfulness.

God, strengthen my hope and renew my strength, and help me to face every challenge with courage and confidence in your faithfulness.

PROJECT IDEA

Creating a Testimony Board

Supplies: **Wooden frame**-the bigger the better, but it can be any size. It *should not* have a glass cover. **Cork** for the background. **Color Paper or Cards**. **Ribbon**. **Decorative Tacks**. **Sheet protectors** for pictures. **Letter Patterns**.

Instructions: Paste the cork to the frame. Use the letters to create the title: **God's Grace in My Life**. It can be placed at the top, at the bottom, or on a side of the frame. Place the ribbon inside following the frame. Any time you experience God's grace in your life, write it down, including the date. It can be typed or handwritten. Attach them to the cork with the decorative tacks. Hang it in your room, office, or anywhere in your house to preserve those moments and be reminded of **God's Grace** in your life.

Day 19 – The Joy of the Soul

"A cheerful heart beautifies the face." – Proverbs 15:13

The joy of the soul is reflected in our whole being. Cultivate joy through gratitude, kindness, and faith in God's promises. True joy springs from a grateful heart and radiates outward, shaping our words, actions, and even our facial expressions. When we nurture joy within, it brightens the days of those around us, becoming a gentle light that draws others closer to the source of our gladness: God. Embrace each day with a spirit of gratitude and let your joy become a testimony to the goodness of God's love.

Lord, fill my heart with joy and allow me to share that joy with those around me. May my life reflect your love and kindness.

PROJECT IDEA

Create a Playlist

Make a list of music and songs that bring happiness and joy to your heart. Create a playlist in your application named "Joyful Sounds" and play it when you are driving or when you feel down.

Day 20 – Joy in Small Actions

"In all things I have taught you that by working in this way, you should help people in need, and remember the words of the Lord Jesus, who said, 'It is more blessed to give than to receive.'" – Acts 20:35

Sometimes we think that to serve we must do great things, but every act of kindness, no matter how small, sows joy in both those who offer it and those who receive it. A smile, a word of encouragement, or an outstretched hand can brighten anyone's day and ignite an inner light in the one who gives it. It is often in gentle, unnoticed acts that true generosity shines. A comforting word, a patient ear, a helping gesture offered without expectation are simple moments that create quiet ripples of joy, reaching farther than we can ever see. Open your heart to serve and discover that small kindnesses weave a tapestry of hope and warmth, blessing both giver and receiver with a sense of connection and purpose.

Lord, help me to cherish the small opportunities to serve and to find joy in every act of kindness I perform.

PROJECT IDEA

Volunteer

Select an organization that speaks to your values and consider volunteering your time. Boys and Girls Clubs are a fantastic option, allowing you to make a difference by mentoring a child. As a mentor, you can share your skills and life experiences, providing guidance and support that can help shape a young person's future. Whether you're helping with homework, leading an art project, or simply being a supportive presence, your time and effort can make a lasting impression.

Day 21 – Service: A Shared Gift

"Let each one according to the gift he has received, minister it to others, as good stewards of the manifold grace of God." – 1 Peter 4:10

Service is not just a favor we give; it is a bridge between souls that transforms both those who help and those who receive. To discover the joy of servicing is to realize that, while bringing well-being to the world, one's heart is filled with meaning and serenity. Embrace the gift of service and find that as you pour out compassion and care, your spirit is quietly replenished with peace and fulfillment. Each time we extend ourselves for another, we step deeper into a purpose that fills our days with quiet joy and lasting contentment. In this journey of service, remain open to the lessons and blessings that come your way. By focusing on the needs of others, you cultivate empathy and understanding, deepening your spiritual growth.

God, teach me to serve with gratitude, seeing every opportunity as a gift to share Your love.

PROJECT IDEA

Food Drive

Organize a food drive in your healthcare unit to create food baskets for low-income patients. Gain support from colleagues and management. Set clear goals for the number of baskets and the needed food items. Concentrate on nutritious non-perishable foods, such as canned vegetables and pasta. Promote the drive through various channels. Set up a convenient drop-off point. Reach out to local businesses for support. After gathering donations, plan a day for volunteers to create personalized baskets with recipe cards. Collaborate with social workers to identify families in need and organize delivery. Stay in touch with participants, show gratitude, and collect feedback to encourage future initiatives, promoting a caring community.

Day 22 – Humility in Service

"And whatever you do, do it from the heart, as unto the Lord and not to people." – Colossians 3:23

Service invites us to recognize other people, with their needs and dreams. In doing so, we learn to see greatness in humility. As one serving the everlasting Father, we must understand that life is never about us, but about Him. It is in that process that joy grows, for nothing elevates the spirit more than giving without expecting a reward. In this journey of service, we discover that true fulfillment lies not in recognition but in the quiet satisfaction of knowing we have touched a life, even in the smallest of ways. Embrace each opportunity to serve with open hearts, finding purpose and joy in every gesture of generosity and love. Be a testament to the power of selfless service, guiding others toward a life of kindness and grace.

Father, may my service always be born from humility and be for Your glory, not seeking recognition but moved by love.

PROJECT IDEA

Set Aside a Day to Honor Key Individuals

Organize a special breakfast or dinner to celebrate housekeeping, environmental services, and food service staff. Engage in meaningful conversations, share stories of their contributions, and express gratitude for their dedication. Consider giving small tokens of appreciation, like personalized notes or certificates. This event fosters community, strengthens relationships, and highlights the importance of recognizing everyone's contributions. Encourage team members to share experiences, promoting a positive and inclusive environment where everyone feels valued and motivated.

Day 23 – The Echo of Generosity

"Give, and it will be given to you; good measure, pressed down, shaken and overflowing, they will give in your lap; for with the same measure with which you measure, they will measure you again." – Luke 6:38

Every time we serve, the joy multiplies. What we generously offer returns in unexpected ways. No act of kindness goes unnoticed. The service we offer is an echo that resonates in people's hearts, reminding us of the power of unity. Like a gentle ripple on still water, each act of kindness we share extends far beyond its source. Service, offered from the heart, becomes a melody of compassion that lingers in the memory of those it touches, inspiring others in turn to give freely and graciously. As you move through your day, let your actions be guided by God's spirit of generosity and compassion, creating ripples of kindness that extend far beyond your immediate surroundings.

Dear God, may my generosity be sincere and abundant, and may I trust that whatever I give out of love, you multiply.

PROJECT IDEA

The Generosity Garden

Create a Generosity Garden in a long-term care facility. A *Generosity Garden* is a community-led project aimed at fostering a culture of giving and teamwork. This initiative involves creating a shared garden where residents can grow fruits, vegetables, and flowers. The harvest will be used to prepare tasty recipes to feed residents, decorate the facility, or be donated to local food banks, shelters, and people in need. This initiative not only advocates sustainable living but also enhances community connections through teamwork and a shared mission.

Day 24 – The Art of Being Present

"Rejoice with those who rejoice; weep with the people who weep." – Romans 12:15

Sometimes, to serve means to be there. Simple. Listen, be present, and share quiet moments. These forms of discreet service open space for deep joy, the joy that springs from knowing that you are useful and connected beyond words. To serve is sometimes holding a hand during uncertainty or quietly observing the light as it shifts across the room. Moments shared in silence are a testament to care that asks for nothing in return. In the art of presence, we discover grace that lingers, asking only that we show up with open hearts and attentive spirits, ready to witness life's joys and sorrows as they unfold. Every silent moment you share is a reminder of the profound impact you have, just by being present. Let this quiet service enrich your spirit and fill your day with a joy that flows from authentic connections and genuine care.

God, give me the sensitivity to be present in the lives of others, and help me to listen without judgment and to accompany with empathy.

PROJECT IDEA

Presence Matters

In today's fast-paced world, the art of being present is often overlooked. Whether it is being there for a friend in need, offering a listening ear, or simply sharing a moment of joy, presence is a powerful gift. This project aims to promote the quality of being present in people's lives, especially during moments of need. Encourage the participation of psychologists, community leaders, or individuals with inspiring stories to join a workshop or seminar, where they can share their insights. Educate participants about the importance of being present and guide how to incorporate this practice into their daily lives.

Day 25 – Pause as a Sacred Act

"I lie down in peace and immediately fall asleep, for you alone, Lord, make me live in confidence." – Psalm 4:8

Pausing, even briefly, is an opportunity to recognize God's presence and find rest amid busy days. These moments of reflection are not just breaks from the physical demands of the day but sacred intervals where your soul finds renewal. It is in these pauses that you rediscover God's rhythm that sustains you. These moments allow you to return to your duties with a refreshed perspective and a heart full of gratitude. Taking a moment to breathe or expressing gratitude is an act of nurturing the soul. In the gentle silence between tasks and worries, we discover a space where peace quietly enters. A moment's stillness allows us to listen to the subtle music of grace and recognize that we are sustained by more than our strength. Invite tranquility and welcome God's presence, allowing your heart to rest and renew.

Lord, bless my pauses and silence; help me sense Your nearness and discover the peace my soul seeks in You.

PRACTICE IDEA

Embrace Stillness

Designate specific times during the day for stillness. Whether it's five minutes in the morning or a mid-afternoon break, consistency is key. Nature is a powerful ally in fostering stillness. Incorporate plants or a small water feature to bring tranquility indoors. Technology can often be a barrier to achieving stillness. Set aside time each day to unplug from screens. Use this time for reading, walking, or simply sitting quietly away from distractions and noise.

Day 26 – Rest amid Service

"Come to me, all who labor and are heavy laden, and I will give you rest."
– Matthew 11:28

In the busy world of hospitals and doctors' offices, it's important to remember that resting can be an act of faith. Resting in God doesn't mean ignoring responsibilities. It means to realize that not everything depends on us. Taking a moment to breathe and pray brings peace that refreshes both body and spirit. Faith invites you to pause, to lay aside the busyness for a moment, and just be. Trust that your life is sustained by grace. Embracing stillness and quietness is an act of courage, an acknowledgment that your worth is not measured by constant motion. Worth is measured by your capacity to trust and receive. As healthcare professionals, embracing these pauses not only benefits our well-being but also enhances the care we provide for others. Allow these pauses to renew your strength. You are never alone on the journey.

Lord, amid daily fatigue, teach me to seek my rest in You, to trust that You sustain every life I care for and mine.

PROJECT IDEA

Promoting Rest in a Healthcare Environment

Host interactive sessions on the benefits of rest for stress management. Set up rooms equipped with comfortable furniture, calming I, and ambient lighting. Develop gardens or outdoor spaces where staff can unwind and enjoy fresh air. Implement rotations that ensure staff have enough downtime between shifts. Recognize team members who emphasize wellness and inspire others to embrace this commitment.

Day 27 – Leaving Burdens in God's Hands

"Cast your burden upon the Lord, and he will sustain you." – Psalm 55:22

Daily, we face uncontrollable situations such as uncertain diagnoses and difficult decisions. Recognizing that we are not alone and finding refuge in God's love helps alleviate unseen burdens. Trusting and surrendering our experiences to God is an act of humility. Entrusting our challenges to God is an act of profound faith. As we release our worries and uncertainties, we open ourselves to God's wisdom and comfort, knowing that our patients will be held by hands far stronger than our own. In the quiet act of surrender, our hearts find renewed peace, and we are reminded that we do not walk this path alone. Invite God's grace to fill the spaces once occupied by anxiety, to restore your spirit, and guide us forward. Embrace the freedom that comes with trusting God's plan, knowing that He holds your future with love and care.

God, I give you my worries, the cases I can't solve, and the people I accompany. May your peace envelop me and give me new strength.

PRACTICE IDEA

Placing Your Trust in God

Engaging in the following practices will help you develop a routine to cultivate a sense of relief and spiritual connection to God. Create a quiet space by finding a comfortable place where you won't be disturbed. Light a candle or play soft, calming music to create a peaceful atmosphere. Spend a few minutes thinking about the burdens that are weighing on you. These could be worries, fears, or emotional pain. Write down each burden on a piece of paper. Be honest and specific about what is troubling you. Pray for guidance and ask for strength and wisdom to let go of what you cannot control. Take a moment to thank God for the support and love you've received. Close in prayer. Repeat daily or weekly.

Day 28 – Renewing the Vocation from Stillness

"In God alone does my soul find rest; from him comes my hope." – Psalm 62:5

To rest in God is to allow one's vocation to be renewed. Service to others requires constant giving, but only those who learn to stop and receive can continue to give. For the joy of serving to flourish again every day, it is necessary to remain connected to God's heart. The burdens we carry become lighter as we surrender them to His care, and the passion that first ignited our hearts is rekindled. True service flows from a heart that finds renewal in quiet moments with God. By pausing to rest in His presence, you allow your strength to be restored and your purpose to be rekindled. Each pause is an invitation to let God refill what selfless giving pours out, ensuring our vocation remains vibrant and rooted in God's love. Let the peace of His presence be the balm that refreshes your spirit and fills you with a renewed sense of purpose.

Dear God, may my vocation be strengthened in your presence. Renew my spirit within your hope and make my service always a reflection of your love.

PROJECT IDEA

Revitalizing Vocation

Organize weekly workshops where employees can learn about and practice quietness techniques. Provide each employee with a personal reflection journal. Encourage your coworkers to spend a few minutes each day jotting down their thoughts, feelings, and any realizations they have about their work and life. Host monthly gatherings where employees can come together to share their experiences and insights gained from the stillness practices. This creates a sense of community and support.

Day 29 – Ever-Present Faithfulness

"Never will I leave you; never will I forsake you." – Hebrews 13:5

When we feel isolated or overwhelmed, God's presence remains constant. In moments of uncertainty, let the assurance of His presence be your refuge. God's presence is not conditional; it is steadfast and unchanging. Regardless of changing circumstances, God's faithfulness remains. He walks beside us in quiet halls, busy workplaces, anxious waiting rooms, and peaceful dawns. We may not always sense His nearness, but His Word assures us we are never abandoned. Let this promise be an anchor for your soul today. When doubt stirs or loneliness whispers, remember you are not alone. Let this promise anchor your soul: God holds you close, offering comfort, guidance, and hope.

Lord, thank you for your unending faithfulness. When I feel alone or unsure, remind me that you never leave or forsake me. Help me rest in your presence and walk forward with renewed confidence, knowing you are always by my side.

PRACTICE IDEA

Reflecting God's Faithfulness

Begin by spending a few quiet moments reflecting on the concept of faithfulness. Consider how God's faithfulness is evident in your life and how it can inspire your actions towards others. Write down your thoughts and insights in your journal. Think about the people in your life who may benefit from an act of kindness or support. Using a calendar or planner, schedule at least three specific acts of kindness you will carry out over the next week. As you carry out each act of kindness, take a moment to reflect on the experience. Consider how it made you feel and how it might have impacted others. Write about these experiences in your journal, noting any insights or emotions that arise. Share your experiences with a group or community, either in a discussion or through social media. Encourage others to participate in similar activities, spreading the message of faithfulness and kindness. Use this opportunity to inspire others to reflect on God's faithfulness in their lives.

Day 30 – His Presence in Every Breath

"The Lord is near to all who call on Him." – Psalm 145:18

In the middle of the demands of daily life, it can be easy to forget that God is always with us. No matter where we are or what we are doing, we can always reach out to Him and feel His presence. Reflect on the constant companionship of Jesus. Whether you are at work, at home, or everywhere else, He is with you, always. Embrace this truth as a source of strength and comfort. His presence brings peace that transcends understanding, offering solace and support when you need it most. Whether it is a whispered prayer in a hectic moment or a quiet reflection in solitude, every encounter with God enriches your spirit and renews your faith. Let the knowledge of His presence inspire you to live with courage and compassion, trusting that He walks with you through every trial and triumph.

Jesus, may each breath I take on this shift become a silent prayer, reminding me that your presence is not limited by place or pace. I know that you are with me always; help me to feel you near and to trust in your constant companionship.

PRACTICE IDEA

In Tune with God

Start a nature walk. Set aside a specific time each week for your nature walk. Early mornings or late afternoons can be especially peaceful. Before you start your walk, take a moment to pray or meditate, inviting God's presence into your time outdoors. This will help you focus and open your heart to the spiritual experience. As you walk, pay close attention to the beauty around you. Notice the colors, sounds, and textures of nature. Consider how these elements reflect the wonder of God's creation. As you walk, take time to reflect on your spiritual journey. If you have a Bible or spiritual text, pause during your walk to read a passage. Reflect on its meaning and how it relates to your life. This practice can deepen your understanding and connection to your faith.

Day 31 – Grace for Every Step

"Your word is a lamp for my feet, a light on my path." – Psalm 119:105

In the journey of life, we often encounter moments of uncertainty and overwhelm. Psalm 119:105 reminds us that God's word is a guiding light, illuminating our path and providing clarity. When we feel lost or burdened, we can turn to His word for direction and comfort. Reflect on the ways God's grace has guided you through challenging times. Each step you take is sacred, and His presence is with you, lighting your way. As you continue your day, remember that every challenge is an opportunity for growth and every decision a chance to align more closely with God's will. Let your heart be a reservoir of peace and joy, filled by the constant flow of God's grace. Trust that you are never alone, for God's light guides you, even in the darkest of moments.

Lord, illuminate my way in this work. When I feel overwhelmed, help me pause and remember that you walk before me, making each step I take in the healthcare world sacred.

PRACTICE IDEA

Cultivating Grace

When in conversation, listen attentively and respond thoughtfully, ensuring the other person feels heard and valued. Regularly reflect on your emotions and their triggers. Journaling can be an excellent tool for this. Put yourself in others' shoes to better understand their feelings and perspectives. Nourish your body with wholesome foods that fuel your energy and enhance your mood. Small gestures, such as holding the door open or offering a compliment, can make a significant impact. Create an environment that promotes calmness by decluttering your space. Regularly thank those around you for their contributions and support.

www.ingramcontent.com/pod-product-compliance
Lightning Source LLC
LaVergne TN
LVHW050939210926
848482LV00013B/671
* 9 7 9 8 3 4 9 5 9 8 0 8 1 *